Probiotic

Dr. Archie E. Perez

What are probiotics?

Probiotics are live microorganisms that are planned to have medical advantages when consumed or applied to the body. They can be tracked down in yogurt and other aged food sources, dietary enhancements, and magnificence items. Instances of serious or deadly contaminations have been accounted for in untimely babies who were given probiotics, and the U.S. Food and Medication Organization (FDA) has cautioned medical services suppliers about this gamble.

In spite of the fact that individuals frequently consider microscopic organisms and different microorganisms destructive "microbes," many are really useful. A few microorganisms assist with processing food, obliterate illness causing cells, or produce nutrients. A large number of the microorganisms in probiotic items are equivalent to or like microorganisms that normally live in our bodies.

Probiotics might contain various microorganisms. The most well-known are microscopic organisms that have a place with bunches called Lactobacillus and

Bifidobacterium. Different microscopic organisms may likewise be utilized as probiotics, thus may yeasts, for example, Saccharomyces boulardii.

Various sorts of probiotics might make various impacts. For instance, assuming a particular sort of Lactobacillus forestalls a disease, that doesn't be guaranteed to imply that one more sort of Lactobacillus or any of the Bifidobacterium probiotics would do exactly the same thing.

Are prebiotics equivalent to probiotics?

No, prebiotics aren't equivalent to probiotics. Prebiotics are nondigestible food parts that specifically invigorate the development or movement of beneficial microorganisms.

What are synbiotics?

Synbiotics are items that join probiotics and prebiotics.

How famous are probiotics?

The 2012 Public Wellbeing Interview Study (NHIS) showed that around 4 million (1.6 percent) U.S. grown-ups had utilized probiotics or prebiotics in the beyond 30 days. Among grown-ups, probiotics or prebiotics were the third most generally utilized dietary enhancement other than nutrients and minerals. The utilization of probiotics by grown-ups quadrupled somewhere in the range of 2007 and 2012. The 2012 NHIS likewise showed that 300,000 kids age 4 to 17 (0.5 percent) had utilized probiotics or prebiotics in the 30 days before the overview.

How should probiotics function?

Probiotics might have various impacts in the body, and various probiotics might act in various ways.

Probiotics may:

Assist your body with keeping a sound local area of microorganisms or assist your body's local area of microorganisms with getting back to a solid condition in the wake of being upset

Produce substances that have positive outcomes

Impact your body's insusceptible reaction.

How are probiotics controlled in the US?

Unofficial law of probiotics in the US is perplexing. Contingent upon a probiotic item's planned use, the FDA could direct it as a dietary enhancement, a food fixing, or a medication.

Numerous probiotics are sold as dietary enhancements, which don't need FDA endorsement before they are advertised. Dietary enhancement marks might make claims about what the item means for the design or capability of the body without FDA endorsement, yet they aren't permitted to make wellbeing claims, for example, saying the enhancement brings down your gamble of getting an illness, without the FDA's assent.

On the off chance that a probiotic will be showcased as a medication for treatment of an infection or confusion, it needs to meet stricter prerequisites. It should be demonstrated protected and compelling for its planned use through clinical preliminaries and be endorsed by the FDA before it tends to be sold.

Finding out About the Microbiome

The people group of microorganisms that lives on us and in us is known as the "microbiome," and it's a hotly debated issue for research. The Human Microbiome Undertaking, upheld by the Public Organizations of Wellbeing (NIH) from 2007 to 2016, assumed a vital part in this exploration by planning the ordinary microorganisms that live in and on the sound human body. With this comprehension of a typical microbiome as the premise, scientists all over the planet, including many upheld by NIH, are presently investigating the connections between changes in the microbiome and different sicknesses. They're additionally growing new restorative methodologies intended to adjust the microbiome to treat sickness and backing wellbeing.

The Public Community for Reciprocal and Integrative Wellbeing (NCCIH) is among the numerous organizations subsidizing research on the microbiome. Specialists upheld by NCCIH are concentrating on the collaborations between parts of food and microorganisms in the gastrointestinal system. The attention is on the manners by which diet-microbiome cooperations might prompt the creation of substances with advantageous wellbeing impacts.

What has science displayed about the adequacy of probiotics for medical issue?

A lot of exploration has been finished on probiotics, however much still needs to be found out about whether they're useful and ok for different medical issue.

Probiotics have shown guarantee for an assortment of wellbeing purposes, including counteraction of anti-toxin related the runs (counting loose bowels brought about by Clostridium difficile), counteraction of necrotizing enterocolitis and sepsis in untimely babies, treatment of newborn child colic, treatment of periodontal illness, and enlistment or support of reduction in ulcerative colitis.

Nonetheless, in many occasions, we actually don't know which probiotics are useful and which are not. We additionally don't have the foggiest idea the amount of the probiotic individuals would need to take or who might be probably going to benefit. In any event, for the circumstances that have been examined the most, scientists are as yet pursuing tracking down the responses to these inquiries.

Probiotics are live microorganisms (organisms) that can usefully affect or inside your body. Each human body is home to trillions of microorganisms that live with us and assist with supporting our physical processes and wellbeing. Not the organisms we might convey are all useful to us — a few kinds (microorganisms) can be hurtful. Yet, gainful organisms, similar to probiotics, help to control the possibly unsafe sorts.

Probiotic items contain select, valuable kinds of microorganisms to add to the populaces previously living in your body. Numerous probiotics are oral enhancements intended to be ingested into your gastrointestinal parcel. Others are effective items that you can apply to your skin or to the mucous films inside your body holes, similar to your nose or privates. There gainful microorganisms usually live.

What do probiotics do?

Probiotics are food and wellbeing items that contribute live, advantageous microorganisms to the populaces inside your stomach and somewhere else, to reinforce those networks. They're intended to forestall and treat dysbiosis — an irregularity or a shortfall of useful microorganisms in your microbiome. At the point when they work, the microorganisms take up home on or in your body, adding to the populaces previously residing there.

However, not all probiotics are similar. Various kinds of microorganisms capability distinctively inside your body, so various sorts may be better or more awful for your condition. Probiotics additionally aren't controlled by the FDA, so makers don't need to demonstrate the quality or even the items in their items. It's really smart to counsel a learned medical services supplier about which probiotics could turn out best for your necessities.

When are probiotics suggested?

In the event that you have side effects of dysbiosis, in your stomach related framework or somewhere else, your medical care supplier could prescribe probiotics to help take your microbiome back to adjust. Assuming you've as of late had an ailment or treatment that debilitated your microbiome, your supplier could propose probiotics to assist with reconstructing it. For instance, they could recommend taking or utilizing probiotics in the wake of following through with a course of anti-toxins.

Certain individuals take an everyday probiotic supplement to keep up with their overall wellbeing. You should do this in the event that you're inclined to destroy medical problems and you notice it makes a difference. A solid stomach microbiome can support your general insusceptibility, decrease irritation and assist with keeping your insides normal. Regular things like pressure and food decisions can decrease your stomach microbiome, and probiotics are one method for reestablishing it.

Which probiotics are powerful?

For a probiotic to have any advantage to your wellbeing, it must:

Be of an assortment that has demonstrated benefits for your body.

Be in a structure that is protected to consume or apply to your body.

Contain reasonable organisms that have endure the business cycle.

Have the option to endure the excursion through your intestinal system (assuming it's an oral probiotic).

Probably the most often examined and suggested probiotics include:

The Lactobacillus family, including L. acidophilus, L. rhamnosus, L. casei and L. plantarum.

The Bifidobacterium family, including Bifidobacterium longum and Bifidobacterium breve.

Acidophilus (L. acidophilus) might be the most notable probiotic available today, potentially on the grounds that it has such countless various applications. Acidophilus is tracked down normally in your mouth, stomach, stomach, lungs, vagina and urinary plot, and it can assist with reestablishing harmony in these microbiomes.

These items are available without a prescription (OTC), in supermarkets, pharmacies and wellbeing and health stores. They come as dietary enhancements (cases, fluids or powders) or as skin salves or creams for various purposes. Your medical care supplier can assist you with choosing a decent one to pursue your necessities.

You can likewise get probiotics in less focused amounts from aged food sources and beverages, including:

Yogurt and kefir.

Curds.

Miso soup.

Fermented tea.

Sauerkraut or kimchi.

Pickles and pickle juice.

Aged food varieties and beverages are one method for getting more probiotics into your GI parcel. Food handling can some of the time obliterate these regular probiotics, however, so actually look at the names for "live and dynamic societies".

Gambles/Advantages

What are the potential medical advantages of probiotics?

The helpful microorganisms that live in various pieces of our bodies help us in different ways. One of the main ways is by fending off the more destructive kinds of microscopic organisms, growths, infections and parasites that could likewise need to live with us. Probiotics, in principle, battle on your gainful organisms.

Numerous probiotic items are figured out with useful microorganisms and yeasts to forestall or recuperating from bacterial or yeast contaminations in your different body parts, including:

Atopic dermatitis and skin break out.

Cavities and gum infection.

Vaginal and urinary plot contaminations (UTIs).

Anti-infection related loose bowels.

Your medical services supplier could recommend utilizing these items preventively on the off chance that you have a background marked by diseases, or utilizing them to assist reestablish your microbiome after therapy with anti-toxins.

Oral probiotics might have numerous extra advantages. Your stomach microbiome — the local area of microorganisms living in your GI parcel — assumes a mind boggling part in your stomach related framework, and in numerous other body frameworks.

Inside your stomach related framework, we know that a sound stomach microbiome:

Helps separate and retain specific supplements and drugs.

Produces other significant supplements as results.

Helps separate and reuse bile after processing.

Helps train your safe framework to perceive and dispense with hurtful organisms.

We likewise know that an undesirable stomach microbiome — one in which destructive microorganisms dwarf the supportive sorts — can add to various persistent gastrointestinal illnesses, including:

Persistent bacterial contaminations like H. pylori and C. difficile.

Little gastrointestinal bacterial excess (SIBO).

Fiery inside illnesses, as ulcerative colitis and Crohn's sickness.

General stomach related hardships, similar to blockage, gas and crabby entrail disorder (IBS).

Taking oral probiotics could help forestall or treat these circumstances, despite the fact that results might fluctuate.

Past your stomach related framework, we know that your stomach microbiome likewise interfaces with your mind and sensory system, your safe framework and your endocrine framework. A few specialists accept that the wellbeing of your stomach microbiome could impact numerous parts of your general wellbeing, including your:

Temperament and agony resilience.

Smartness and exhaustion.

Aggravation and resistant reaction.

Digestion, glucose and fat stockpiling.

However, this is all still under dynamic examination. We don't completely comprehend how everything functions yet, or what impacts probiotics could have inside these body frameworks, if any. There's insufficient proof to make strong inferences, but rather there's enough for some medical services suppliers to suggest attempting them.

Are there any dangers or incidental effects to taking probiotics?

While there's little unambiguous examination on the security of probiotics, they give off an impression of being ok for sound individuals to take. They have a long history of far reaching and ordinary use among general society. There's a little gamble of unfavorable secondary effects for individuals with more fragile invulnerable frameworks. This incorporates individuals taking immunosuppressant drugs, individuals with basic ailments and newborn children who've been conceived rashly.

The gamble is that a probiotic item could contain a destructive kind of microorganism alongside the supportive sorts. Microorganisms are tiny, so it's feasible for some unacceptable kind to sneak through unnoticed in the event that an item isn't thoroughly tried. This is interesting, and it's anything but a significant gamble for the vast majority. A sound safe framework will effortlessly get out the fraud. However, in a debilitated safe framework, it could cause a serious contamination.

Extra Normal Inquiries

How might I let know if probiotics are working for me?

On the off chance that you're taking probiotics for a particular reason, and the probiotics are working, you ought to have the option to tell that you're feeling much improved. For instance, assuming you're taking them to assist with easing obstruction or looseness of the bowels, you ought to see your craps turning out to be more managed after some time. In the event that you're taking them to ease a bacterial or yeast disease or excess, you ought to see your side effects getting to the next level.

Ensure you're taking them reliably, and at the suggested measurements, so you can appropriately decide how well they're functioning. In the event that you're taking them preventively, it very well may be more enthusiastically to tell. For instance, certain individuals take probiotics to work on their invulnerability during the cold and influenza season. You could see that you haven't been wiped out as frequently to no one's surprise, yet it's difficult to be aware in the event that that is because of the probiotics.

Could probiotics at any point cause loose bowels, blockage or stomach torment?

Many individuals take probiotics to assist with easing the runs, blockage or stomach torment. Over the long haul, probiotics ought to further develop your general stomach wellbeing, including your inside consistency and absorption, decreasing distress. In any case, temporarily, conceivable presenting new probiotics could set off comparable side effects, particularly in the event that you're taking an enormous portion or on the other hand assuming that your stomach will in general be delicate overall.

Numerous probiotics produce a result called short-chain unsaturated fats in your stomach. These results have many advantages to your stomach wellbeing, however an unexpected deluge of them could cause transitory loose bowels. Different probiotics produce gases in your stomach as side-effects. Assuming you abruptly have a greater amount of them than expected, you could see expanded swelling and gas during processing. These side effects ought to determine inside a couple of days.

What's the most ideal way to take probiotics?

You can accept probiotics as a dietary enhancement, or you can help them through matured food varieties and beverages. There are advantages to the two techniques. As a rule, food and drink sources could assist with advancing a more noteworthy variety of organisms in your biome, which is really great for keeping up with your overall wellbeing. Some food sources may likewise incorporate prebiotics, the filaments that probiotics need to benefit from to flourish.

To treat a specific issue, you should take a particular probiotic supplement that your medical care supplier has suggested for that reason. An enhancement will regularly give a higher portion of probiotics than food sources will. Accept it as suggested on the mark. A few probiotics work better with food, and others while starving. Most should be taken everyday for the best outcomes.

A note from Cleveland Center

There's a ton of examination underway on the possible advantages of probiotics, and introductory outcomes are promising. Different probiotic items might assist with further developing your skin wellbeing, your vaginal wellbeing or your stomach wellbeing and develop your resistance overall. While they may not be the complete answer for your medical problems, they could give a significant piece of the riddle. Get some information about taking probiotics. They can assist you with picking the best one for you, guarantee your wellbeing and screen your outcomes.

How Would They Function?

Specialists are attempting to sort out precisely the way in which probiotics work. A portion of the manners in which they might keep you solid:

At the point when you lose "great" microbes in your body, for instance after you take anti-toxins, probiotics can assist with supplanting them.

They can help balance your "great" and "terrible" microorganisms to keep your body working the manner in which it ought to.

Kinds of Probiotics

Many kinds of microbes are delegated probiotics. They all have various advantages, however generally come from two gatherings. Get some information about which could best assistance you.

Lactobacillus. This might be the most widely recognized probiotic. It's the one you'll track down in yogurt and other aged food varieties. Various strains can assist with looseness of the bowels and may assist with peopling who can't process lactose, the sugar in milk.

Bifidobacterium. You can track down it in some dairy items. It might assist with facilitating the side effects of bad tempered entrail disorder (IBS) and another circumstances.

Saccharomyces boulardii is a yeast tracked down in probiotics. It seems to assist with battling loose bowels and other stomach related issues. This is what to search for while picking the best probiotic for ladies and men.

What Do They Do?

In addition to other things, probiotics assist with sending food through your stomach by influencing nerves that control stomach development. Analysts are as yet attempting to sort out which are best for specific medical conditions. A few normal circumstances they treat are:

Bad tempered inside condition

Incendiary gut sickness (IBD)

Irresistible loose bowels (brought about by infections, microorganisms, or parasites)

The runs brought about by anti-toxins

There is additionally some exploration that shows they're helpful for issues in different pieces of your body. For instance, certain individuals say they have assisted with:

Skin conditions, similar to dermatitis

Urinary and vaginal wellbeing

Forestalling sensitivities and colds

Oral wellbeing

Instructions to Utilize Them Securely

The FDA controls probiotics like food, dislike drugs. Dissimilar to tranquilize organizations, creators of probiotic supplements don't need to show their items are protected or that they work.

Inquire as to whether taking probiotics is smart for you. As a general rule, probiotic food sources and enhancements are believed to be ok for the vast majority, however certain individuals with insusceptible framework issues or other serious medical issue shouldn't accept them.

At times, gentle secondary effects could incorporate a furious stomach, looseness of the bowels, gas, and swelling for the primary two or three days after you begin taking them. They may likewise set off hypersensitive responses. Quit taking them and converse with your PCP in the event that you have issues.

Things to be aware of probiotics

Unofficial law of probiotics in the US is mind boggling. Contingent upon a probiotic item's planned use, the US Food and Medication Organization (FDA) could manage them as a dietary enhancement, a food fixing, or a medication.

Numerous probiotics are sold as dietary enhancements, which don't need FDA endorsement before they are advertised. Food sources with live or dynamic societies are separated structure probiotics.

Live or dynamic societies models:

Any food with maturation microbe(s)

Verification of reasonability at any rate level intelligent of average levels seen in matured food varieties is recommended being 1×109 CFU per serving

No particular examination or proof is expected to make this case.

Probiotics standards for items that don't make a wellbeing guarantee:

A member(s) of a protected animal types, which is upheld by adequate proof of an overall helpful impact in people or a safe microbe(s) with a property (for instance, a construction, movement, or final result) for which there is adequate proof for an overall useful impact in people

Verification of feasibility at the fitting level utilized in supporting human examinations

Probiotics measures for items that make a wellbeing guarantee:

Characterized probiotic strain(s)

Verification of conveyance of reasonable strain(s) at an effective portion toward the finish of time span of usability

Persuading proof required for explicit strain(s) or strain mix in the predetermined wellbeing sign

Our body regularly has our idea of good or supportive microbes and terrible or hurtful microorganisms. Keeping up with the right harmony between these microscopic organisms is important for ideal wellbeing. Age, hereditary qualities, and diet might impact the arrangement of the microorganisms in the body (microbiota). An unevenness is called dysbiosis, and this has potential connects to illnesses of the digestive system, including ulcerative colitis, crabby inside condition, celiac infection, and Crohn's sickness, as well as additional foundational sicknesses like stoutness and type 1 and types 2 diabetes. How can you say whether you really want probiotics? This article will assist you with choosing.

What are prebiotics and synbiotics?

The prebiotic precedes and helps the probiotic, and afterward the two can consolidate to make a synergistic difference, known as synbiotics. A prebiotic is really a nondigestible carb that goes about as nourishment for the probiotics and microbes in your stomach. The meaning of the impact of prebiotics is the particular feeling of development as well as activity(ies) of one or a set number of the microbial genus(era)/species in the stomach microbiota that confer(s) medical advantages to the host. The medical advantages have been recommended to incorporate going about as a solution for gastrointestinal (GI) intricacies like enteritis, blockage, and bad tempered gut sickness; counteraction and therapy of different tumors; diminishing unfavorably susceptible irritation; therapy of nonalcoholic greasy liver infection (NAFLD), and battle invulnerable lack illnesses. There has likewise been research showing that the dietary admission of specific food items with a prebiotic impact has been shown, particularly in young people, yet additionally probably in postmenopausal ladies, to increment calcium retention as well as bone calcium growth and bone mineral thickness.

The advantages for stoutness and type 2 diabetes are developing as late information, both from exploratory models and from human examinations, have shown specific food items with prebiotics have impacts on energy homeostasis, satiety guideline, and body weight gain.

The majority of the prebiotics distinguished are oligosaccharides. They are impervious to the human stomach related proteins that work on any remaining sugars. This implies that they go through the upper GI framework without being processed. They then, at that point, get aged in the lower colon and produce short-chain unsaturated fats that will then feed the valuable microbiota that lives there. Oligosaccharides can be combined or gotten from regular sources. These sources incorporate asparagus, artichoke, bamboo shoots, banana, grain, chicory, leeks, garlic, honey, lentils, milk, mustards, onion, rye, soybean, and sugar beet, sugarcane juice, tomato, wheat, and yacón. The medical advantages of these oligosaccharides are a subject of continuous exploration.

What are microorganisms and their part in our wellbeing?

Microorganisms are minuscule organic entities (microbes, infections, parasites, or growths) - - so little that millions can squeeze into the opening of a needle - - that are strong to such an extent that an irregularity in the body is connected with various illnesses. These microorganisms can be tracked down in pretty much all aspects of the human body, living on the skin, in the nose, and in the stomach. There are trillions of these microorganisms in our bodies. They dwarf human cells by 10 to one, yet because of their little size, they just make up 1%-3% of a body's complete mass.

The Human Microbiome Venture, upheld by the Public Organizations of Wellbeing (NIH) from 2007 to 2016, assumed a vital part in examination into the bacterial piece of the body by planning the ordinary microorganisms that live in and on the solid human body. With this comprehension of a typical microbiome as the premise, scientists all over the planet, including many upheld by

NIH, are currently investigating the connections between changes in the microbiome and different illnesses.

What are the medical advantages of probiotics?

Probiotics might appear new to the food and supplement industry, however they have been with us from our most memorable breath. During a conveyance through the birth waterway, an infant gets the microbes Bacteroides, Bifidobacterium, Lactobacillus, and Escherichia coli from his/her mom. These great microscopic organisms are not sent when a Cesarean segment is performed and have been demonstrated to be the justification for why a few babies brought into the world by C-segment have sensitivities, not exactly ideal insusceptible frameworks, and lower levels of stomach microflora.

What precisely do probiotics do? They are accepted to safeguard us in two ways.

The first is the job that they play in our assimilation. We realize that our gastrointestinal system needs a good overall arrangement among great and terrible stomach microbes, so what impedes this?

It appears as though our way of life is both the issue and the arrangement. Unfortunate food decisions, profound pressure, absence of rest, anti-microbial abuse, different medications, and ecological impacts can all move the equilibrium for the terrible microorganisms.

Medical advantages of probiotics

At the point when the gastrointestinal system is solid, it sift through and disposes of things that can harm it, like destructive microbes, poisons, synthetic compounds, and other byproducts. The good arrangement of microbes helps with the guideline of gastrointestinal motility and upkeep of stomach obstruction capability. Research has shown a few advantages for the utilization of probiotics for irresistible looseness of the bowels, anti-infection related the runs, stomach travel, IBS, stomach torment and bulging, ulcerative colitis, Helicobacter pylori contamination, nonalcoholic greasy liver illness (NAFLD), and necrotizing enterocolitis.

The alternate way that probiotics help is the effect that they have on our safe framework. Some accept that this job is the most significant. Our resistant framework is our insurance against microorganisms. At the point when it doesn't work as expected, we can experience the ill effects of unfavorably susceptible responses, immune system issues (for instance, ulcerative colitis, Crohn's sickness, and rheumatoid joint inflammation), and diseases (for instance, irresistible the runs, H. pylori, skin contaminations, and vaginal diseases). By keeping up with the right equilibrium from birth, the expectation is forestall these diseases. Our resistant framework can benefit whenever that decent is reestablished, so it's rarely past the point of no return.

Examination into the advantages of probiotics has been fanning out, and new regions are arising. Starter research has connected them to supporting the wellbeing of the conceptive parcel, oral depression, lungs, skin, and the stomach mind hub, and the anticipation and treatment of heftiness and type 1 and type 2 diabetes.

Sorts of probiotics: Lactobacillus

Probiotic enhancements, food sources, and refreshments contain microbes and additionally yeasts. Up until the 1960s, the main stomach microflora that they had the option to recognize were clostridia, lactobacilli, enterococci, and E. coli. From that point forward, imaginative methods have found a lot more microorganisms.

There are a few various types of probiotics, and their medical not set in stone by the gig that they do in the stomach. They should be recognized by their sort, species, and probiotic strain level. Here is a rundown of probiotics and their conceivable medical advantages.

1. Lactobacillus

There are in excess of 50 types of lactobacilli. They are normally viewed as in the stomach related, urinary, and genital frameworks. Food sources that are aged, similar to yogurt, and dietary enhancements additionally contain these microbes. Lactobacillus has been utilized for treating and forestalling a wide assortment of sicknesses and conditions.

A portion of the lactobacilli found in food varieties and enhancements are Lactobacillus acidophilus, L. acidophilus DDS-1, Lactobacillus bulgaricus, Lactobacillus rhamnosus GG, Lactobacillus plantarium, Lactobacillus reuteri, Lactobacillus salivarius, Lactobacillus casei, Lactobacillus johnsonii, and Lactobacillus gasseri.

Studies have shown a few advantages connected to Lactobacillus and treating or potentially forestalling yeast contaminations, bacterial vaginosis, urinary plot disease, crabby inside condition, anti-infection related loose bowels, voyager's the runs, loose bowels coming about because of Clostridium difficile, treating lactose prejudice, skin issues (fever rankles, dermatitis, skin inflammation, and ulcer), and counteraction of respiratory diseases.

Sorts of probiotics: Bifidobacteria

2. Bifidobacteria

There are roughly 30 types of bifidobacteria. They make up the majority of the sound microbes in the colon. They show up in the digestive system not long after birth, particularly in breastfed babies, and are believed to be the best marker of gastrointestinal wellbeing.

A portion of the bifidobacteria utilized as probiotics are Bifidobacterium bifidum, Bifidobacterium lactis, Bifidobacterium longum, Bifidobacterium breve, Bifidobacterium infantis, Bifidobacterium thermophilum, and Bifidobacterium pseudolongum.

Studies have shown that bifidobacteria can assist with further developing blood lipids and glucose resistance. Bifidobacteria have been displayed to really reduce IBS and fundamentally further develop IBS side effects like agony/distress, distension/bulging, desperation, and stomach related messes.

Sorts of probiotics: Saccharomyces boulardii, Streptococcus thermophilus, Enterococcus faecium, Leuconostoc

3. Saccharomyces boulardii

This is otherwise called S. boulardii and is the main yeast probiotic. A few examinations have shown that it is compelling in forestalling and treating the runs related with the utilization of anti-microbials and explorer's looseness of the bowels. It has additionally been accounted for to forestall the reoccurrence of C. difficile, treat skin break out, and lessen the results of treatment for H. pylori.

4. Streptococcus thermophilus

This produces enormous amounts of the compound lactase, making it successful, as per a few reports, in the counteraction of lactose bigotry.

5. Enterococcus faecium

This is ordinarily tracked down in the digestive system of people and creatures.

6. Leuconostoc

This has been utilized broadly in food handling all through mankind's set of experiences, and ingestion of food sources containing live microbes, dead microscopic organisms, and metabolites of these microorganisms has occurred for quite a while.

Food varieties with the most probiotics: Kefir

The revelation of the advantages of probiotics started with sharp milk. Today we have numerous different choices to get different microscopic organisms from our food sources, in spite of the fact that it's not quite so straightforward as adding them to the food. For there to be medical advantages, the microorganism must have the option to endure the section through the gastrointestinal plot, endure the food fabricating process, and develop and get by during the aging or stockpiling period. Likewise, the microorganisms should not adversely influence item quality and be remembered for the By and large Perceived as Protected (GRAS) list.

Most microorganisms are remembered for the maturation interaction. Maturation broadens the time span of usability of short-lived food varieties. It is a sluggish decay interaction of natural substances prompted by microorganisms or catalysts that basically convert sugars to alcohols or natural acids. The lactic corrosive supplies the microorganisms that then add medical advantages to the food. You can buy food varieties that are aged or mature them yourself.

Kefir: This could be the best probiotic dairy item since it contains the two microorganisms and yeast cooperating to give various medical advantages. In a new eight-week study, individuals with diabetes were given kefir milk containing Lactobacillus casei, Lactobacillus acidophilus, and bifidobacteria versus regular matured milk. The hemoglobin A1C levels were altogether lower in the gathering consuming the kefir.

Food sources with the most probiotics: Kimchi

Kimchi: This aged vegetable is produced using Chinese cabbage (beachu), radish, green onion, red pepper powder, garlic, ginger, and matured fish (jeotgal). Numerous microorganisms have been viewed as present and can incorporate any of the accompanying: Leuconostoc mesenteroides and Lactobacillus plantarum,

L. mesenteroides, L. citreum, L. gasicomitatum, L. brevis, L. curvatus, L. plantarum, L. sakei, L. lactis, Pediococcus pentosaceus, Weissella confusa, and W. koreensis. A new survey connected the medical advantages of kimchi to anticancer, antiobesity, anticonstipation, colon wellbeing advancement, cholesterol decrease, antioxidative and antiaging properties, mind wellbeing advancement, insusceptible advancement, and skin wellbeing advancement.

Food varieties with the most probiotics: Yogurt, Sweet acidophilus milk, Different food varieties

Yogurt: It can contain Streptococcus thermophilus, Lactobacillus bulgaricus, L. acidophilus, and Bifidobacterium bifidum. Research has shown joins with yogurt to emphatically affect the stomach microbiota and is related with a diminished gamble for gastrointestinal illness and improvement of lactose prejudice (particularly among youngsters), type 2 diabetes, cardiovascular infection, sensitivities, and respiratory sicknesses, as well as worked on dental and bone wellbeing.

Sweet acidophilus milk: L. acidophilus and L. acidophilus in addition to bifidobacteria are added to make this milk.

Different food varieties without significant exploration: miso (aged soybean glue); tempeh; sauerkraut; matured delicate cheddar; sourdough bread; sharp pickles; gundruk (nonsalted, aged, and acidic vegetable item); sinki (native matured radish tap root food); khalpi (aged cucumber); inziangsang (conventional matured verdant vegetable item ready from mustard leaves); soidonis (broad aged item ready from the tip of mature bamboo shoots)

What are the secondary effects and dangers of probiotics?

Supplements assume a significant part when the eating routine isn't sufficient to supply our necessities. On account of probiotics, one's eating routine is the best hotspot for probiotics. These are live microscopic organisms and should be painstakingly observed, put away, and consolidated for the medical advantages that one would be taking them for. As referenced beforehand, contingent upon a probiotic item's expected use, the FDA could control it as a dietary enhancement, a food fixing, or a medication. Numerous probiotics are sold as dietary enhancements, which don't need FDA endorsement.

There is one Deliberate Certificate Program by which an enhancement producer can decide to be assessed. ConsumerLab.com (CL) is the main supplier of free experimental outcomes and data to assist purchasers and medical services experts with distinguishing the best quality wellbeing and sustenance items. Items that have passed their testing for character, strength, virtue, and breaking down can print the CL Endorsement on their item. This is one stage toward being sure that one is getting the sum and sort of probiotic guaranteed by the producer.

Alert should be taken by each and every individual who decides to take these enhancements, however this is particularly valid for kids, pregnant ladies, old endlessly individuals with compromised invulnerable frameworks. For individuals with compromised safe frameworks because of illness or therapy for an infection (like disease chemotherapy), taking probiotics may really build one's possibilities becoming ill. It has been shown that the utilization of different probiotics for immunocompromised patients or patients with a defective stomach has brought about contaminations and sepsis (disease of the circulatory system). One instance of bacteremia (microbes in the circulation system) was as of late found when somebody with dynamic extreme provocative entrail sicknesses with mucosal disturbance was given Lactobacillus GG. Continuously talk with a specialist prior to taking any enhancement under these conditions.

* 9 7 9 8 8 7 1 1 3 0 3 9 1 *